CARB CYCLING MADE EASY FOR WEIGHT LOSS

The Ultimate Guide to Foolproof 7-Day Weight Loss Plan

OLANREWAJU SOYOMBO

Legal Disclaimer

The information presented here is not intended to guarantee any automatic result or any guarantee as to how fast the result will come.

It is your responsibility to proceed with caution and do your due diligence before proceeding with any advice included in this eBook.

The author/publisher will not assume any liability or be held responsible for any financial loss, injury, or personal loss. There are risks involved with anything relating to life and body improvements, and you assume all such risks and waive any responsibility to the Author/publisher.

Results will vary from person to person, and there is no guarantee that any specific results to be made.

Table of Contents

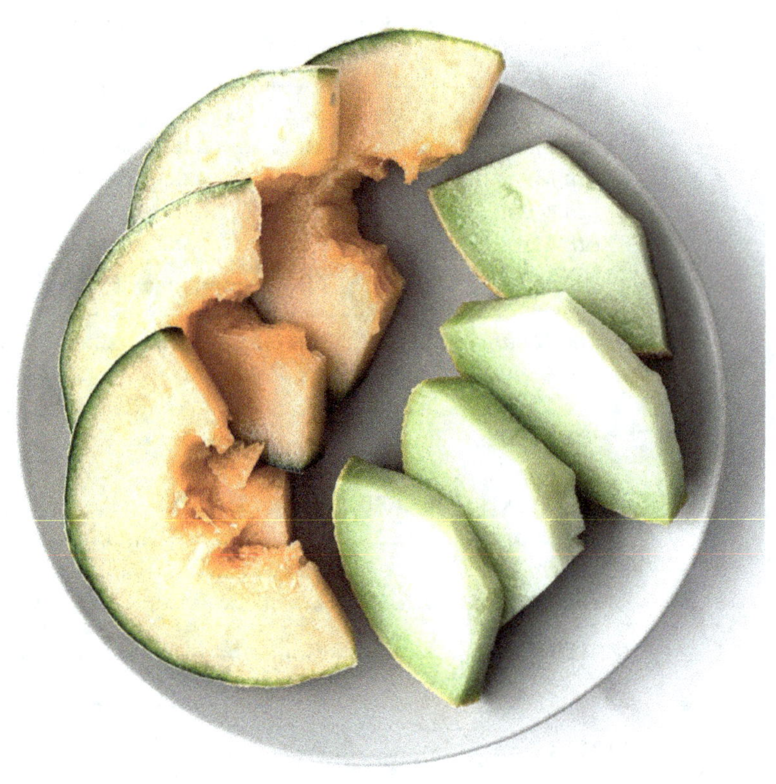

Introduction

The term "carbs" (Carbohydrates) is tantamount to sacrilege for anyone attempting to lose weight. Carbohydrate is the age-old foe. Carbohydrates are the plague of every Weight Watcher. Carbs equal calories, and weight loss necessitates calorie reduction.

This was the old idea that eating foods high in carbs would cause you to gain weight. Carbs are abundant in even good carbohydrates like starchy vegetables and entire grains. Therefore many traditional diets restrict them. As a result, we've evolved to assume that carbs are hazardous to our health. They not only obstruct weight reduction, but they are also quite harmful.

In recent years, research has flipped this notion on its head, claiming that carbs might be your best partner in reducing weight. Carb cycling is the process of using carbs to help us lose weight. This is one way carbohydrate consumption might contribute to weight loss rather than gain!

Carb cycling is accomplished by following a weekly meal plan with fundamental guidelines. Apart from that, you get to eat whatever you want. Your favorite healthy foods, including carbs, may be included in your meal plans. You even have days when you cheat and eat your favorite less-nutritious meals to satisfy your cravings!

What sets the 7-day plan apart?

Many of us battle weight and want to be healthy and fit. We've all tried a variety of diets. We tried diets that claimed dramatic weight loss in a short period. We tried diets that claimed we'd never be hungry or tired again. We tried regimens that said you could eat anything you wanted and still lose weight, only to discover that "everything" only meant half a teaspoon.

We've been let down several times. Either we fall off the wagon and begin to shiver uncontrollably or get too disheartened to continue. Most, if not all, traditional diets could be more effective for humans.

What distinguishes the carb cycling strategy? To begin with, it makes sense because it focuses on our metabolism rather than our stomach. After all, our metabolism burns calories and helps us lose weight.

Second, while it has lately been heralded as a breakthrough in healthy eating and weight reduction, it has long been popular among athletes, particularly those who engage in high-resistance exercise. Carbohydrate cycling is used by many of them to grow lean muscle and boost their energy levels.

Finally, a carb recycling plan is less stringent than other diets. This makes it simple to understand. The strategy should only be utilized to attain short-term weight loss objectives, after which you should cease.

You may, however, use parts of it to create good lifetime eating habits that will help you stay fit and healthy for the rest of your life.

This is a step-by-step tutorial for those who wish to attempt the 7-day carb cycling diet for the first time. We won't get into the nitty-gritty of how carb recycling works, the several hormones it activates, or tough measures.

It will explain how and why carb cycling works and what you'll need to do to put your 7-day carb cycling plan together. The outcomes will be self-evident.

So, if you're considering the carb cycling diet, this book will get you started. But I'll have to include the standard disclaimer here. Consult your doctor before beginning this plan if you have a chronic condition or are taking any medications.

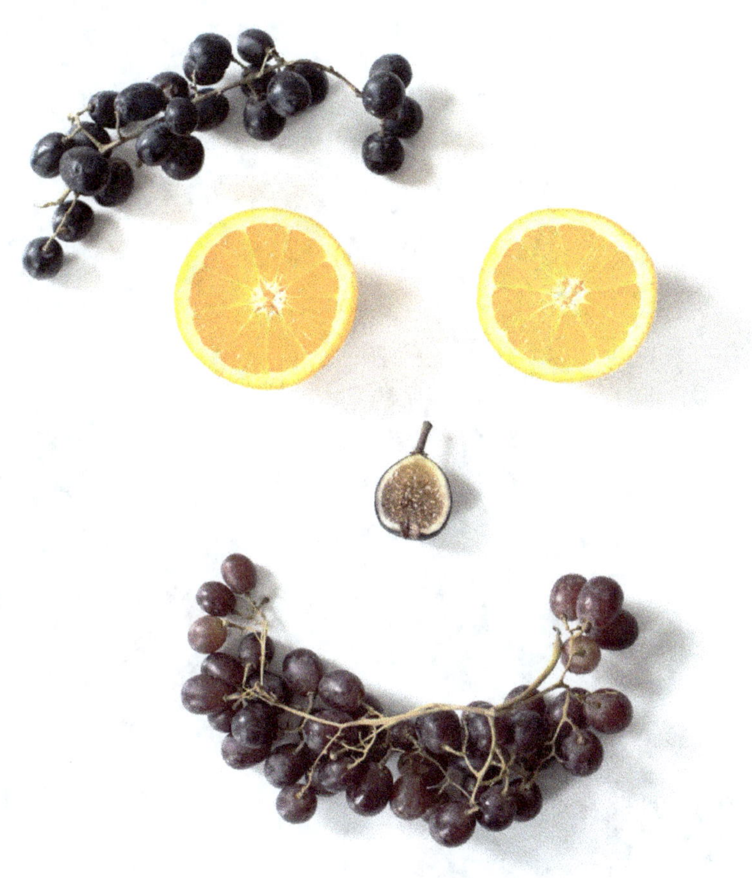

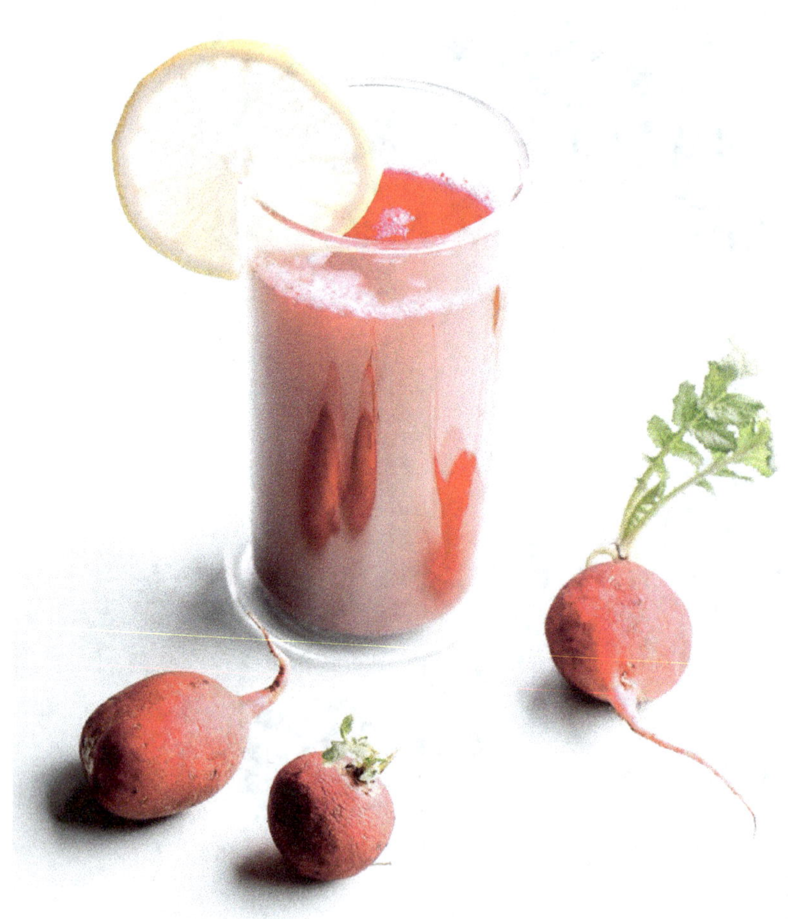

Chapter 1

Carb Cycling: How It Works

Do you recall how ancient railway trains used to operate? Workers had to shovel massive amounts of coal into an enormous coal furnace. The train would continue to run at full speed if the furnace was fueled regularly. The train's speed would be reduced if the coal intake was reduced. The train would only halt if the furnace were constantly replenished with coal.

The metabolism of our bodies works similarly. Carbohydrates are the primary dietary category that "fuels" our metabolism, allowing it to burn calories and provide us with energy. Carbohydrates are also a good source of energy. As a result, diets that eliminate or severely restrict carb consumption leave us weary and sluggish. They make us irritated, hungry, and more prone to binge eating.

A person follows the 7-day carb cycling strategy to improve their metabolism. The diet encourages the body to employ carb-rich meals to perform at its best, burning fat and gaining muscle. As a consequence, you'll lose weight while gaining less fat. It's that straightforward! This is what distinguishes carb cycling as revolutionary.

However, there is a catch. This does not imply that you should go crazy with carbohydrates and eat them daily. The caveat is that you have to stick to a seven-day schedule in which you consume more carbohydrates on some days and less or no carbs on others. This helps your body to "cycle" your carb consumption in the most efficient way possible, allowing you to lose weight and gain muscle mass.

The reasoning is that your body is forced to burn fat for energy when your carb intake is low, and your fat intake is high. This is what leads you to lose weight. High-carb days aim to keep your metabolism fueled and operating at its best, giving you energy.

What Does The 7-Day Plan Entail?

The weekly diet alternates high-carb days with low-carb days to maintain your metabolism in a normal fat-burning cycle.

You may raise your carb consumption while lowering your fat intake on high-carb days. You can eat tiny amounts of carbohydrates or avoid them entirely on low-carb days while boosting your fat and protein intake.

Athletes and frequent exercisers generally time their high-carb days with practice or exercises when their energy levels peak. You should think about it for days when you're very active.

Example of a standard 7-day plan

Monday: Lots of carbs. Tuesday: Carbohydrate restriction Wednesday is a carb-heavy day. Thursday is a low-carb day. On Friday, eat a lot of carbs.

Saturday: Carbohydrate-heavy day – or a chance to treat yourself. You can eat everything you want (in moderation). This is often referred to as "cheat day." Sunday is a carb-free day.

The 7-day plan in many forms

Various diet variants include two or more high-carb days followed by two or more low-carb days or a variation of this. Here are a few examples:

1st Alternative Plan

Day 1: Lots of carbs

Day 2: Carbohydrates are limited.

Day 3: There will be no carbs.

Day 4: Carbohydrates are limited.

Day 5: Carbohydrates abound

Day 6: Carbohydrates are limited.

Day 7: There will be no carbs.

2nd Alternative Plan:

Day 1: Lots of carbs

Day 2: Carbohydrates are limited.

Day 3: There will be no carbs.

Day 4: Carbohydrates are limited.

Day 5: Carbohydrates

Day 6: Carbohydrates are limited.

Day 7: There will be no carbs.

Other versions include four days of high carb followed by three days of low carb. However, as a novice, you should start with a simple, alternate-day plan.

When you feel ready, you can transition to a different cycle. Alternatively, you can continue the simple regimen until you reach your weight loss target.

Consider these other choices if carb cycling is a good fit for you. In this case, you should seek expert assistance. They'll collaborate with you to develop a plan specific to your weight reduction objectives, gender, and lifestyle.

We'll utilize the alternate-day schedule because it's the easiest for the beginning and will work for everyone.

The Food You Eat

Carbohydrates: Carbs are the body's primary fuel source and are required for metabolism to function correctly. They're also necessary for kicking-starting the fat-burning cycle.

Protein is the cornerstone of a successful carb cycling strategy. With each meal, you must consume around 1/5th to 1/7th of the daily minimum need.

Fats: Throughout the program, your fat consumption will be steady. On low-carb days, you should increase your fat consumption somewhat to boost your energy.

Measuring your daily consumption

Calculate your daily carbohydrate, protein, and fat intake for the most significant outcomes. This is a reasonably simple multiplication procedure.

Days with a low-carb intake

Carbs: Double a woman's body weight by 0.6. Bodyweight should be multiplied by 0.9 for men. The final figure represents your daily carbohydrate intake in grams.

Proteins: By multiplying their body weight by 1.2, women may determine their daily consumption. Men's daily consumption may be calculated by multiplying their body weight by 1.5. The resultant figure will be the daily protein consumption needed.

Fats: Women should multiply their body weight by 0.5, while males should multiply by 0.8 to determine daily fat consumption. The resultant value represents your daily fat consumption in grams.

Add the totals from the three food groups to get the total number of calories.

Days with a lot of carbs

The identical formula is performed; only your carbohydrate and protein consumption will be more significant in this scenario. The amount of fat you consume will decrease.

Carbs: Women's body weight should be multiplied by 1.4, while men's should be multiplied by 1.7.

Proteins: Women's body weight is multiplied by 1.4, while men's body weight is multiplied by 1.7 (yep, it's the same ratio as carbohydrates).

Women's body weight should be multiplied by 0.3, while men's should be multiplied by 0.6.

Add the three figures together for high-carb days to get the total number of calories you can ingest.

It is entirely up to you how you divide your daily consumption between meals, whether you eat three or six times a day.

Calories

Women should consume 1500–2300 calories daily, whereas males should consume 1500–3000 calories daily. This is the overall suggested range in which you should stay. Don't be too hard on yourself if you go overboard on certain days. I strongly advise you to get a calorie counter app.

You can find out how many calories are in your food items by looking them up online and making a reference list on your computer.

Quantity

On high-carb days, carb amounts vary from 200 to 300 grams, whereas on low-carb days, carb portions range from 50 to 150 grams. In a subsequent chapter, we'll talk about quantities and food kinds.

This was a quick rundown of how the carb-cycling diet works. Let's examine why it works and how it may help you.

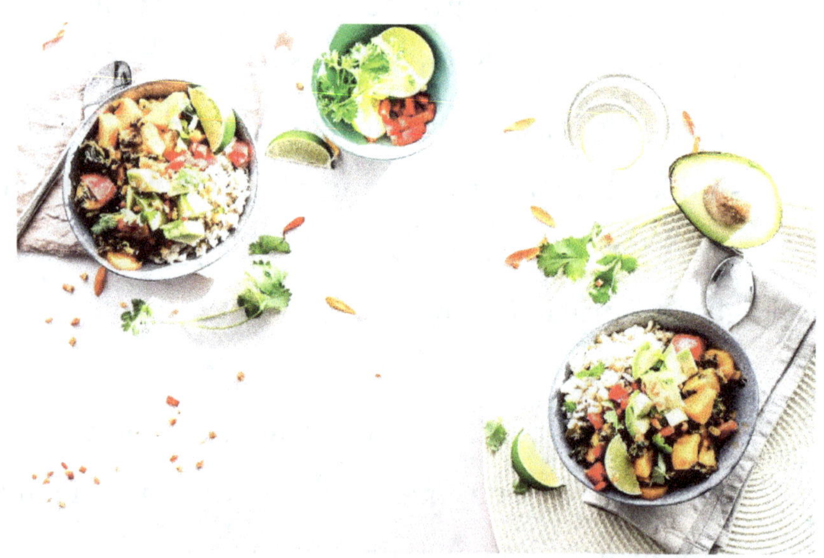

Chapter 2

The Benefits of the Carb Cycling Diet

The carb-cycling diet has lately gained popularity. In terms of the extra advantages, research is still underway.

However, many people have experienced excellent success with the 7-day regimen for various reasons. The following are some of the reasons why it works:

- Flexibility is one of the most critical factors. There is a broad range of meals to pick from, so it doesn't feel like a diet. On some days, you are allowed to consume your favorite meals. People that stick to the diet say they don't feel deprived. In addition, the cheat day is beneficial!

- If you follow the fundamental guidelines, you can personalize your strategy.

- It's simple to include in your daily routine and become a permanent or long-term dietary habit.

- It's a straightforward procedure. Anyone who wants to reduce weight may easily follow the simple instructions.

- Perhaps the most compelling feature is that it has been shown to build muscle and burn fat simultaneously. This is a once-in-a-lifetime opportunity for anyone looking to lose weight.

- A high-carbohydrate diet has been proven to enhance pancreatic insulin production. This essential hormone aids in the acceleration of metabolism and the production of energy. Insulin also aids in the maintenance of healthy body composition.

- A high carbohydrate diet boosts leptin synthesis, a hunger-suppressing hormone.

- High-carb days will replenish and fuel glycogen, a muscle-building chemical.

- You don't need to track macronutrients or use strict measures. Simply keeping track of your daily calorie consumption and adhering to the fundamental rules can provide benefits.

It was formerly thought that you couldn't grow muscle and reduce fat simultaneously. This is because lowering weight necessitates a lower calorie consumption while developing power necessitates a higher calorie intake.

Carb cycling, miraculously, is the secret recipe that allows the body to accomplish both. This is a game-changer.

Carb cycling is practical since it is a healthy approach to losing weight and improving fitness.

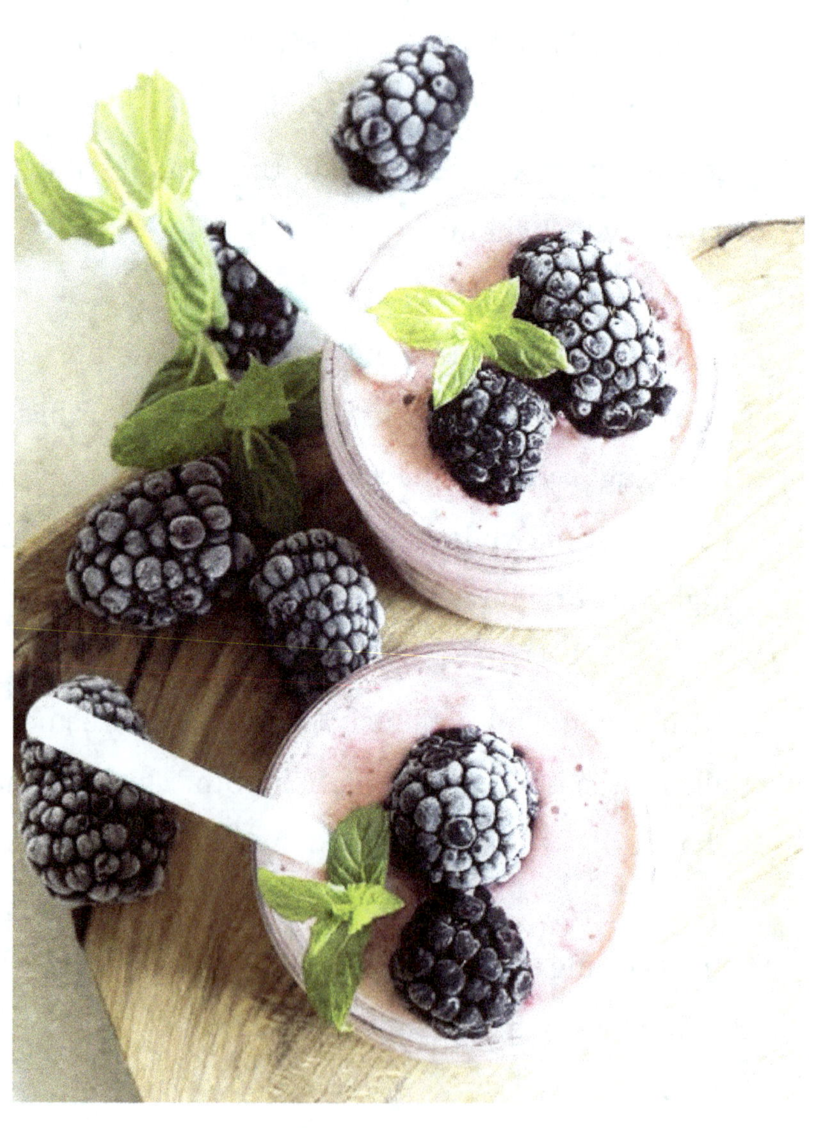

Chapter 3

Making a Good First Impression

Planning ahead of time will save you a lot of time, trouble, and blunders. Here are the fundamentals you'll need to start on the right foot.

Select a Strategy

To begin, determine which days will be the high carb and which will be low carb. We'll follow the alternating high-carb/low-carb day schedule for simplicity after the meal plans to match your days if you want to utilize another of the abovementioned variations.

It's ideal if your high-carb days coincide with your most active days, but this is only sometimes the case. Choose your "cheat day" next.

This is the strategy you'll follow over the following month. Switching plans during a cycle is not suggested since it will break the current process.

Make up Your Mind on the Number of Meals to Prepare

It's entirely up to you how many meals you consume every day. Instead of the traditional three meals, some people prefer four to six smaller meals. This diet could suit you if you're used to nibbling more during the day.

The three-meal programs also include healthful snacks. If you're the sort of person who gets hungry frequently, eating multiple meals each day will help.

More advanced carb cyclers may use fasting or eat only two meals a day. This is not, however, a good idea for novices.

Make a Meal Plan for the Week

This is the most enjoyable part! If you're genuinely organized, you should schedule your meals weekly, bimonthly, or monthly. This will save you the time and effort of assembling a dinner at the last minute.

The day, whether high- or low-carb, and the number of meals should be listed on the meal plan.

Each meal should be preceded by the time you want to consume it. The epochs are only a guideline. When you're hungry, you can eat your next meal sooner.

There will also be days when you cannot keep to your routine. You can eat your meals later but skip them entirely to avoid being dehydrated.

Ensure You Have Enough Food

All of the items for your meal plans should be in your cupboards and refrigerator. Weekly shopping for all of your food requirements is a brilliant idea. Some meals can be frozen; others can be stored, ensuring the vegetables do not spoil. In a subsequent chapter, you'll receive sample meal plans to help you.

Remember to stick to your selected plan for at least four weeks before switching between high and low-carb days.

Stock Up on Healthy Carbs That Will Last a Long Time

Potatoes, almonds, and legumes are just a few examples of nutritious carbohydrates with a lengthy shelf-life. Purchase in large quantities to ensure that you never run out of carbohydrates.

Food portions that are recommended

Some meal plans contain portions in half-cups or cups, in addition to calorie and gram consumption and suggested carbohydrate amounts (if you are using meal plans you found online, for example). This is entirely OK. Complicated conversions are unnecessary.

You'll notice that your fat and protein consumption will be higher on low-carb days. Make sure you're getting enough healthy fats and proteins in your diet.

Invest in a compact food scale to quickly measure amounts in grams and ounces. The appropriate daily carbohydrate, protein, and fat consumption should be followed.

DAYS WITH A LOT OF CARBS

TYPE OF FOOD	PER POUND OF BODY WEIGHT IN GRAMS
Carbs	2–2.5 gm.
Proteins	1 gm.
Fats	0 -0.15 gm.-

DAYS WITH LOW CARB

Once you've established these foundations, you're ready to go on to the next step: **deciding what to consume and avoid.**

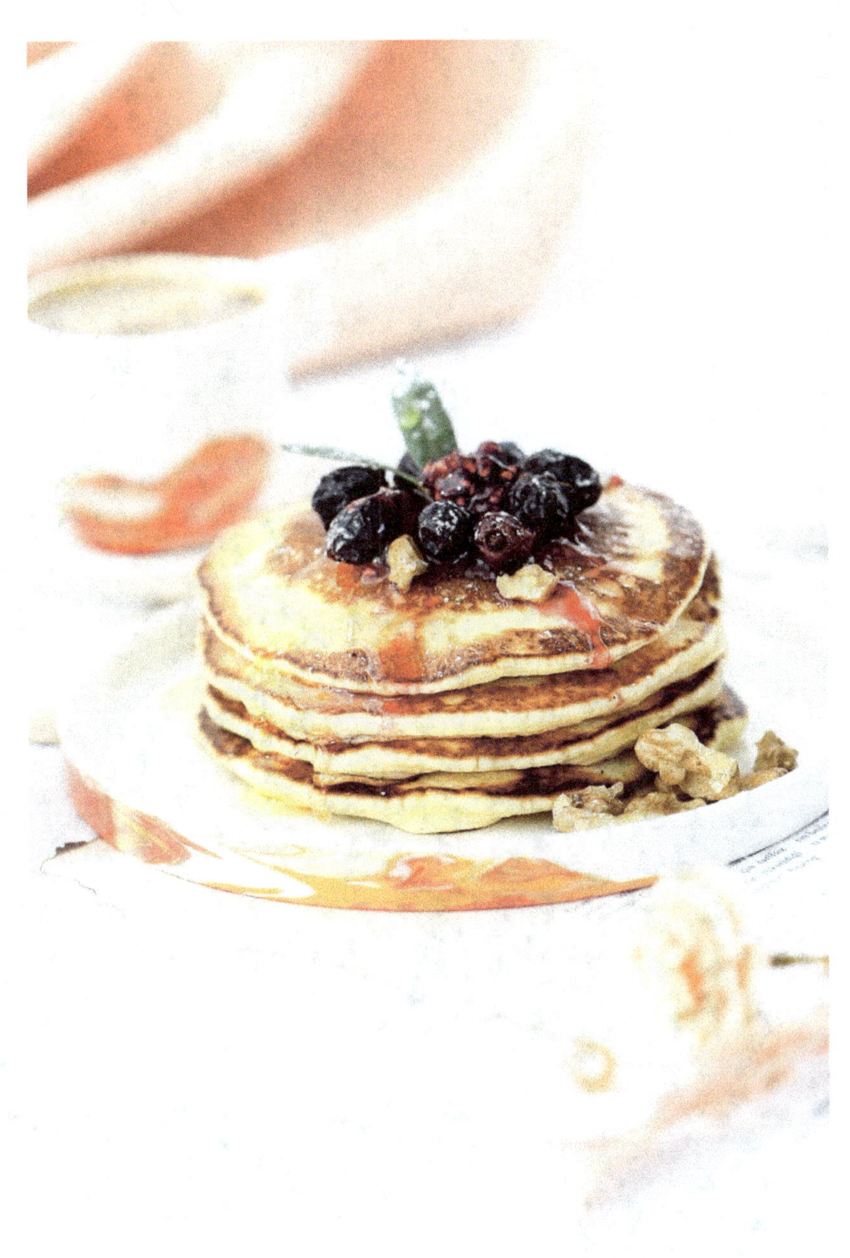

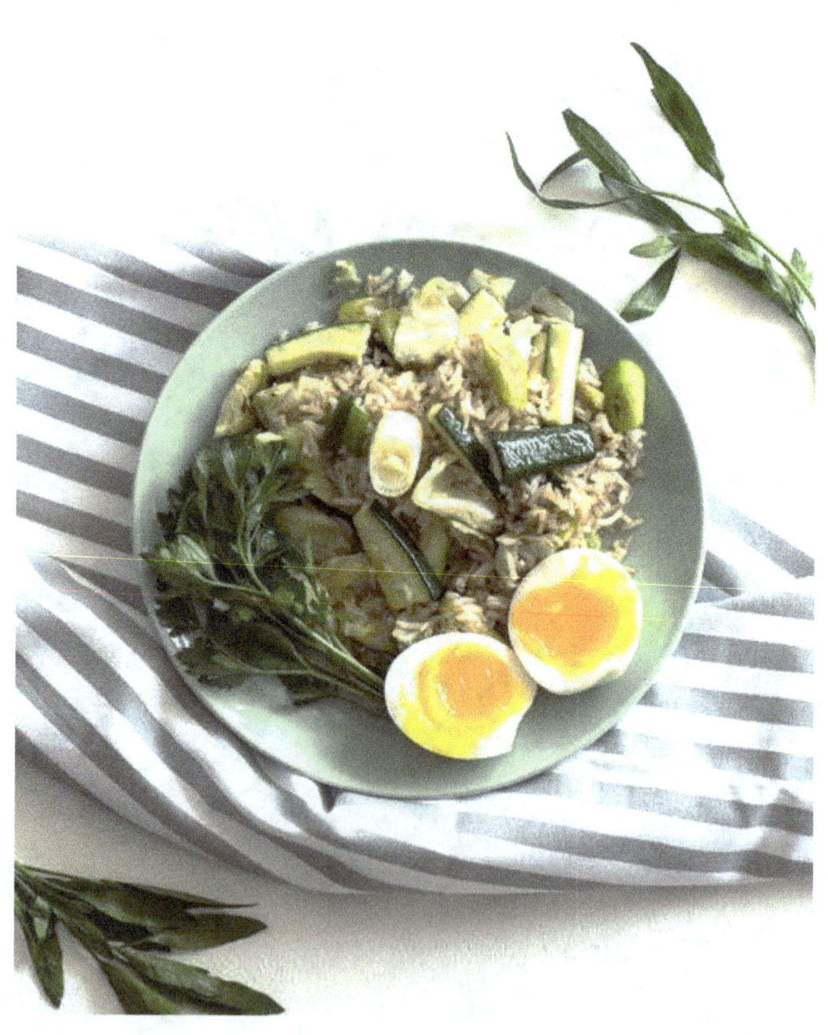

Chapter 4

What to Eat and What to Stay Away From

Good vs. Bad Carbs

First and foremost, you must consume healthy carbs and avoid bad carbs at all costs. Complex or unprocessed carbohydrates are healthy carbs. Processed carbohydrates are the ones that are high in empty calories and have little nutritional value.

This is one of the essential restrictions to follow if you want your carb plan to function. So, if you're hooked on white bread, muster the courage to abstain from it except for one piece on cheat days. Fortunately, there is something for everyone on the list of nutritious carbs.

GOOD UNPROCESSED CARBS	BAD COMPLEX CARBS
Brown rice	White or whole wheat flour
Natural sweeteners like honey or molasses	Table sugar
Whole grain bread	Processed cereals
Whole grain pasta	Store-bought cookies and cakes
Sprouted grains like buckwheat, oats, and quinoa	Soft drinks
White potatoes	Pizza
Sweet potatoes	French fries
Lentils	white pasta
All types of beans and legumes	Muffins
Butternut squash	Tortillas and wraps
Oatmeal	Processed chips and similar snacks
Corn	Ice cream

Peas	Jams and jellies
Couscous	Processed fruit juices
Fruits rich in carbs like Bananas, peaches, plum Pineapple, and blueberries	Bagels and pretzels
Beets	Chocolate and Candy
Some vegetables with low amounts of carbs include tomatoes, mushrooms, cabbage, Brussel sprouts, and peppers.	Pancakes
Dates	Beer

Good vs. Bad Fats and Proteins

Vegetables, proteins, and fats are the basis of your low-carb days. But if you're eating unhealthy fats and proteins on low-carb days, that defeats the purpose. Healthy fats and proteins boost the process of carb cycling and give you more energy. Make sure you include a good variety of these in your plan.

HEALTHY DAYS AND PROTEINS FOR LOW CARB DAYS	UNHEALTHY FATS AND PROTEINS
Grass-fed lean meat	Processed like meats bacon, and pastrami luncheon meats
Organic eggs	Hot dogs and sausage
Poultry	
Fish, especially that high in healthy Omega-3 fats like tuna, salmon, and mackerel	Heavy cream and milk
Raw dairy products like goat cheese, feta, and ricotta	Peanut butter

Low-fat dairy products	
Nuts and seeds	
Olive oil, palm oil, and coconut oil	
Leafy greens and all non-starchy vegetables	
Avocados	
Apples and apricots	
Almond butter	

It would be best if you now had a good sense of what I'm talking about. You can now start carb cycling by incorporating healthful foods into your meals.

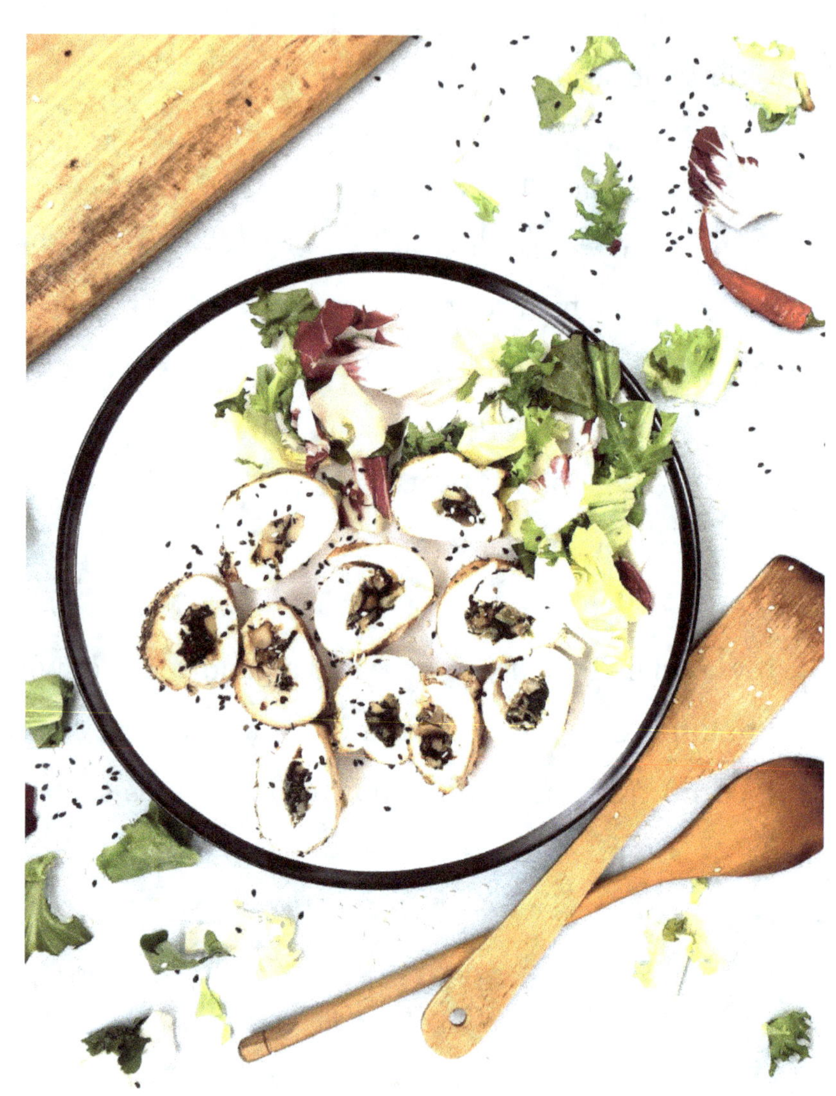

Chapter 5

Meal Plan Examples

Putting this information into a meal plan might require more work for novices. These meal ideas for an average carb cycling week should be of assistance.

Use them as a starting point for meal planning, but remember that they aren't set in stone. Depending on your 7-day plan, you can add or remove meals.

1st PLAN

Monday (a day with low carb)

Breakfast

- 3 scrambled, poached, boiled, or fried whole eggs
- 1/2 cup high-carb fruit (blueberries, pineapple, or peaches, for example)
- 1 cup honey-sweetened oatmeal

Snack

- 1/2 cup unsalted nuts or 1 apple

Lunch

- Turkey sandwich on whole-wheat bread with lettuce and tomato
- Herbal tea

Snack

- 2 medium apricots or 1/2 cup ricotta cheese

Dinner

- Frittata de Spinach
- Beef strips grilled with green bell peppers
- Salad Verde

Tuesday (a day with high carb)

Breakfast

- Swiss cheese on two pieces of whole wheat bread
- 1 cup fresh blueberries in low-fat yogurt

Snack

- 1 banana

Lunch

- Brown rice with grilled salmon
- Salad with grated carrots and cucumbers

Snack

- 1 whole wheat slice with almond butter

Dinner

- Pasta made with whole wheat and fresh tomatoes
- Garlic-infused black beans
- A healthy green salad

Wednesday (a day with low carb)

Breakfast

- 3 avocado-topped scrambled eggs

Snack

- 2 plums or 2 apricots

Lunch

- Grilled chicken pieces in a Caesar salad
- Tea made from natural ingredients

Snack

- 1/2 cup of nuts or low-fat yogurt

Dinner

- Green beans and onions with a flank steak
- Feta cheese in a green salad

Thursday (a day with high carbs)

Breakfast

- 2 whole-wheat toast slices
- 1/2 pound of fruit
- 2 eggs poached

Snack

- 1 banana or 1/2 cup fruit or nuts

Lunch

- Sweet Potatoes

- Salad Verde

- A cup of brown rice laced with chickpeas

Snack

- 1 banana or low-fat yogurt with honey

Dinner

- Chicken breasts on the grill

- Salad with tomatoes and avocados

- Potato, baked

Friday (a day with low carb)

Breakfast

- a half-cup of oats

- 1/2 pound of fruit

- 1/2 cup ricotta cheese, feta cheese, or goat

cheese

Snack

- 1 low-fat yogurt or 1/2 cup fruit or nuts

Lunch

- Salad with avocado and chicken
- Tomato slices on lettuce
- Tea made from herbs

Snack

- An orange, an apple, or two plums

Dinner

- Vegetables and grilled salmon
- Pilled Beans
- Salad Verde

Saturday (a day with high carb)

Breakfast

- Whole-wheat toast bread with 2 scrambled eggs

- 1 honey-sweetened low-fat yogurt

Lunch

- Lentil soup
- Sweet potatoes

Snack

- A half-cup of nuts or fruit

Dinner

- Whole wheat noodle tuna casserole
- Salad with spinach

Sunday (minimal carb + cheat day)

Breakfast

- Fried eggs with lean sausages
- Fruit (1/2 cup)

Snack

- 1/2 cup of nuts or almond butter

Lunch

- Salad with tuna

- 1 fresh fruit slice

Snack

- 1 apple, 2 plums, or 2 apricots

Dinner:

You can do whatever you want! Please use caution. For example, order two instead of two or three slices of pizza. Allow yourself a small amount of ice cream or cake. If you've been craving French fries all week, serve yourself a modest dish rather than a large platter. You get my drift.

2nd PLAN

Here is a sample meal plan to help you if you eat more than three meals daily.

AN EXAMPLE OF A LOW-CARB DAY

1st Meal

- 3 eggs
- 3 lean bacon slices
- Peppers sautéed

2nd Meal

- Grilled turkey or chicken breast (4 oz.)
- 1 carrot cup
- Salad with lettuce and tomatoes

3rd Meal

- 4 oz. salmon, tuna, or shrimp to grill
- 1 pound broccoli
- A single banana

4th Meal

- Chicken (4 oz.)

- 1 pound of spinach

- 1 tablespoon honeyed low-fat yogurt

5th Meal

- Tuna (4 oz.)
- 1 cup chickpeas
- 1 sliced cucumber or tomato

6th Meal

- Lean steak (4 oz.)
- Lean steak (4 oz.)
- 1/2 cup of fruits

AN EXAMPLE OF A HIGH-CARB DAY

1st Meal

- 2 eggs
- 3 bacon strips or 3 tiny sausages
- 2 slices of whole-wheat toast bread

2nd Meal

- 4 oz. chicken
- Green salad
- 1/2 cup honeyed oatmeal

3rd Meal

- Salmon (4 oz.)
- 1/2 cup of brown rice
- 1/2 cup of peas and carrots

4th Meal

- 1 cup arb-rich fruit such as peaches, plums, or

apricots

- 4 oz. chicken

- 2 cups spinach

5th Meal

- 1 cup of corn

- 1 cucumber slice

- 1/2 cup wild rice or quinoa

6th Meal

- Grilled beef steak (4 oz.)

- 1 yam

- 1 cup green beans

- Green salad

Lunch

- 1 piece of a whole fruit

- Green salad

- Lean ground beef tacos

OR…

- Stuffed bell peppers with lean minced beef
- Cucumber and spinach slices topped with grated Parmesan cheese
- 1 apple

OR…

- Lettuce-based chicken salad
- Herb-baked butternut squash

Dinner

- Honey-sweetened oatmeal
- Carrot and green beans
- Whole wheat spaghetti with grilled chicken pieces and Parmesan cheese

OR…

- Jelly cup

- Salad of shredded lettuce and tomato

- Beef stroganoff with mushrooms

OR...

- Chicken fajita wraps

- 1 piece of whole fruit

- Stuffed zucchini boats with mozzarella

DAYS OF EXTREME CARB

Breakfast

- Bacon and chives scrambled eggs
- Honeyed oats with blueberries
- 1 whole fruit piece

OR...

- Scrambled eggs
- Cream cheese on 2 slices of whole-wheat bread
- A single banana

OR...

• Sausage with fried eggs

• 2 whole pieces of toast

• 1 yam

Lunch

• Turkey sandwich on a grilled bun

• Salad with chickpeas

• Honeyed yogurt

OR...

• Salmon on the grill

• Salad with sweet potatoes and spinach

• 1 whole fruit piece

OR...

• Whole-wheat noodle dish with shrimp

• Salad with potatoes

• 1 whole fruit piece

Dinner:

- 1 piece whole fruit
- Baked chicken
- Peas with carrots

OR...

- Pan-fried steak with potatoes
- Sweet corm broccoli
- Jelly cup

OR...

- Chicken and mushroom pasta
- Salad with cherry tomatoes and spinach
- Honeyed quinoa

As you can see, there's plenty of room to be inventive and come up with delectable dishes. Once you've mastered it, you'll be able to whip up delicious delights for the entire family to enjoy (but non-plan family members and children should be open to quantities and calories).

You can also make your favorite dishes carb-cycling-friendly by substituting healthy carbohydrates for processed carbs and saturated fats for beneficial fats.

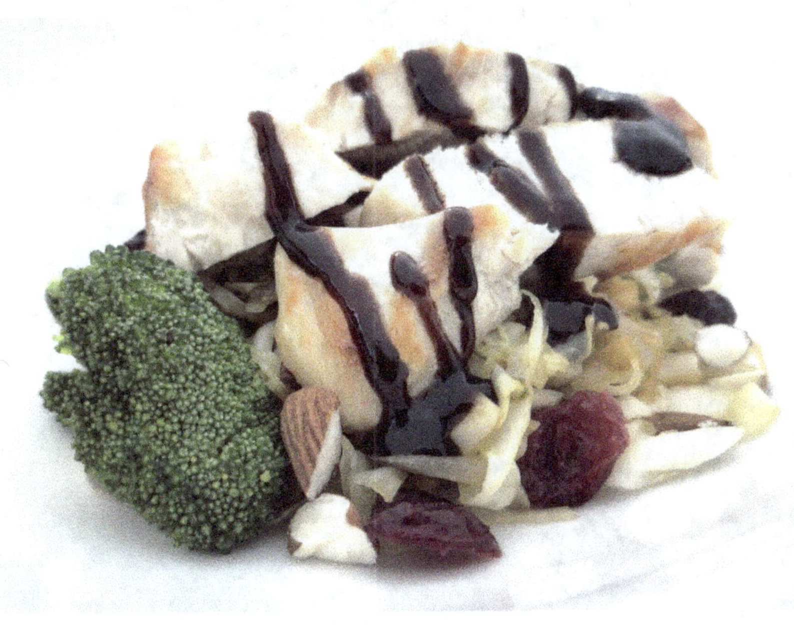

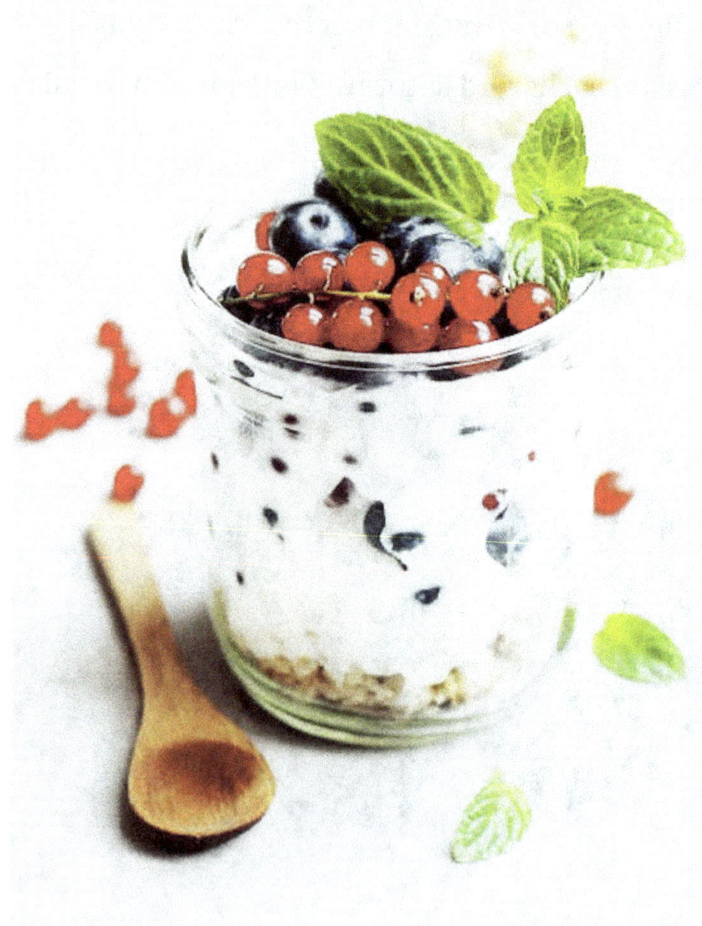

Chapter 6

Expected Common Side Effects

Don't be concerned. The side effects aren't even close to becoming harmful. Consider them to be mild signs and symptoms that may cause pain.

Any abrupt dietary or activity modifications may result in some transient adverse effects. It's similar to when you get back into shape after a long period of inactivity. After that, your muscles will hurt for a few days. However, you are aware that it is a result of your training.

Some persons who started the carb cycling regimen have complained of adverse effects. Within a week or two, they should be gone or considerably reduced.

1. Weight increases due to water. Expect to gain some water weight, especially when you eat a lot of carbs. This is because your body stores four times more

water for every gram of carbohydrates you ingest. Over time, this should return to normal.

On low-carb days, you'll observe less water weight gain. So don't worry; you're not gaining weight.

Exercising on days when you eat a lot of carbs may also assist. Note: Even if you gain weight due to water retention, you should continue drinking enough water throughout the day.

2. During the first week, you may feel more fatigued and sluggish than usual. This is very normal. Once the carb cycling sets in, you'll restore your average energy — in fact, you'll feel an increase in power.

3. You may suffer from bloating or constipation. You eat many carbs, especially starchy meals like potatoes and rice.

Herbal drinks, particularly chamomile, are an excellent remedy for this. You may substitute your fruit consumption with stewed fruit until your digestion recovers.

4. You could be irritated and have mood changes. This is a prevalent issue. The carb cycling strategy may need to be more relaxed for you. What exactly does that imply?

   You're limiting yourself if you're used to consuming more carbohydrates than the amounts recommended in this diet. For the first several days, this deprivation may induce irritation and moodiness.

5. Switching from harmful carbohydrates and fats to healthy carbs and fats may cause cravings. You'll be able to conquer this with the assistance of willpower and a cheat day.

6. On low-carb days, your body may want more carbohydrates.

There is no significant danger in following a carb-cycling diet other than the above-mentioned mild side effects. Always pay attention to what your body is telling you.

The carb diet may not suit you if you experience these adverse effects for over two weeks.

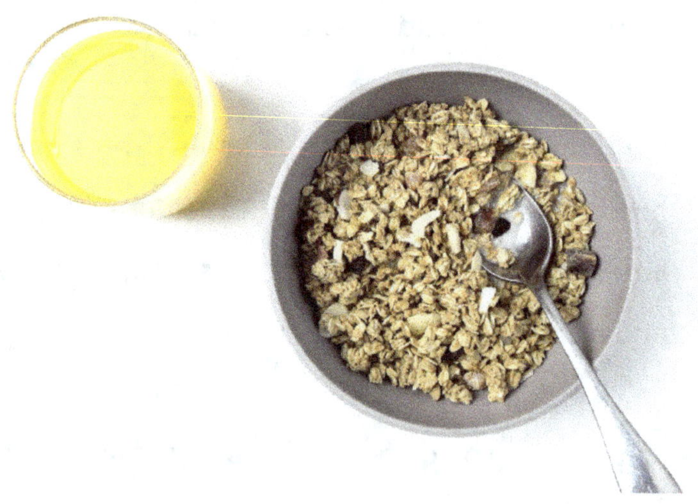

Chapter 7

Recommendations

Here are some helpful hints to help you improve the effectiveness of your carb-cycling diet. Some of these you may already be doing.

1. Cheat days are not an open invitation to gorge yourself on your favorite foods. If you're starving, get a slice of pizza or a Big Mac. Remember that a cheat day is an option, not a must.

   How often you "cheat" affects your carb cycling outcomes. Of course, if you do it once a week, your weight reduction will be slower. Keep cheat days to a minimum if you want faster results.

2. Eat breakfast and always include protein and fiber in your diet. This is crucial for staving off hunger pangs and keeping you full until your next meal.

3. Consider resistance or aerobic training to keep your muscle mass and make the most of carb cycling. Any exercise will be suitable if this is something other than your thing. Walking, riding, and swimming are all viable options.

4. If you participate in sports or work out regularly, time your high-carb days with your high-activity days. This will assist you in losing weight more quickly. Additionally, you will have more energy on such days.

5. Do not consume calories by "drinking" them. Examples are smoothies, sweetened tea, coffee, and fruit juices. Stay hydrated with water or herbal tea. If you must have coffee in the morning, try to drink it black. When it comes to tea, when it's sweetened with honey, it's pretty decent.

6. Supplements can help you keep your carb cycling in check and aid your digestion. Probiotics, omega-3 fatty acids, and vitamin B12 are all acceptable alternatives.

7. Be inventive when it comes to food planning. Work with the many items you have on hand to make delectable recipes. Look for new recipes to try online and experiment with different carb combinations.

   Also, try new foods like quinoa, kale, or hummus that you've never eaten before. It's possible that you'll be pleasantly surprised!

8. Get adequate rest to be energized and stress-free. Allow your body to rest to achieve optimum carb cycling. For anyone looking to improve their health, this is simple basic sense.

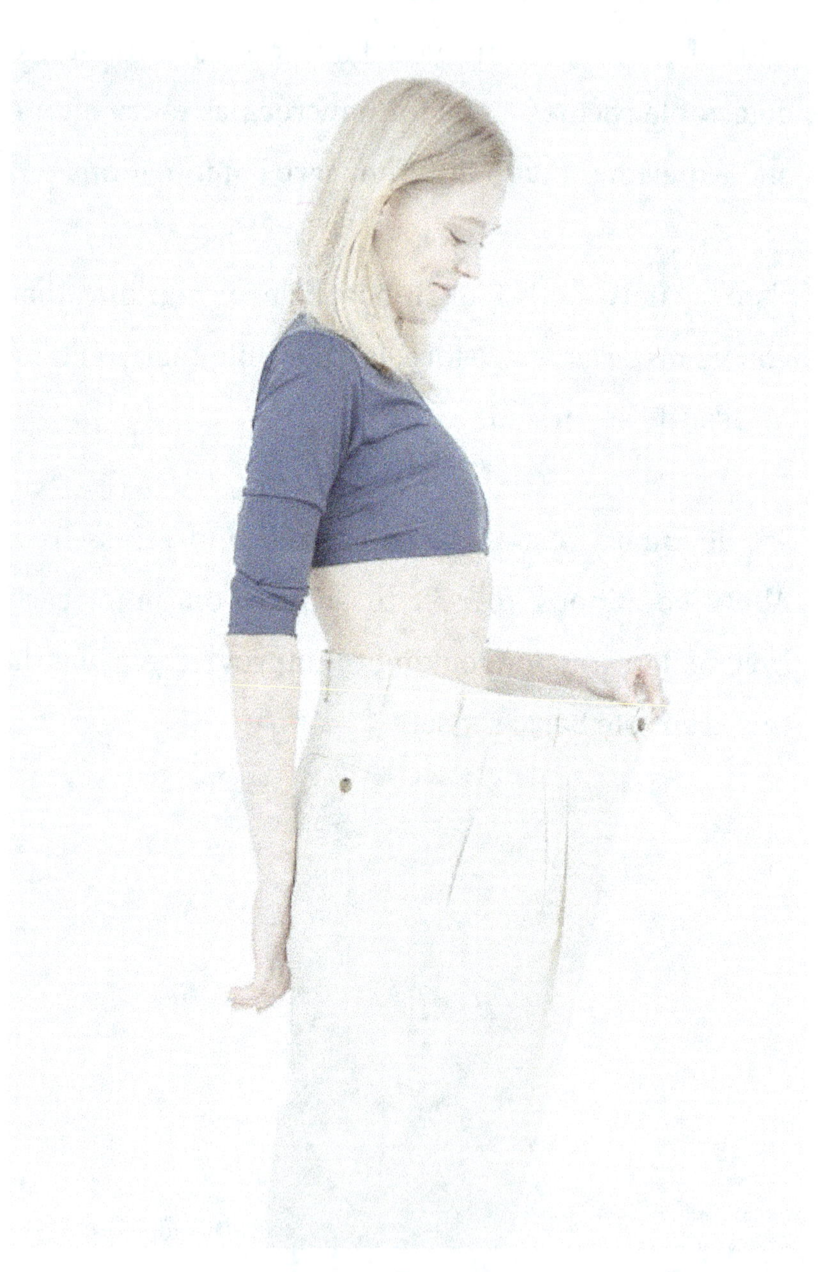

Conclusion

This was a straightforward explanation of how the carb diet works. We've gone over everything you need to know to get started.

So, what are the main points to remember?

- Carb cycling works by simultaneously burning fat and building muscle by fueling your metabolism.

- Carb cycling is a 7-day plan alternating between high and low-carb days.

- You base your meals on the recommended daily carbohydrate, protein, and fat intake.

- You shed pounds!

Carbohydrate-free diets do not work for everyone.

Deprivation and the resulting cravings can be overwhelming.

You'll have a much better chance of sticking to the 7-day carb cycling plan because it's not restrictive. You can still eat carbs even if you're on a low-carb diet. This may be the most straightforward and least painful way to shed pounds.

It's worth a shot if you like the versatility and variety of foods. People have reported that it is far less rigid and restricting and that they rarely feel hungry. Of course, losing weight while increasing muscle mass is the ultimate benefit.

So go ahead and stock up on healthy carbohydrates and proteins, have fun with your meal plans, and start looking, feeling, and getting in shape today.

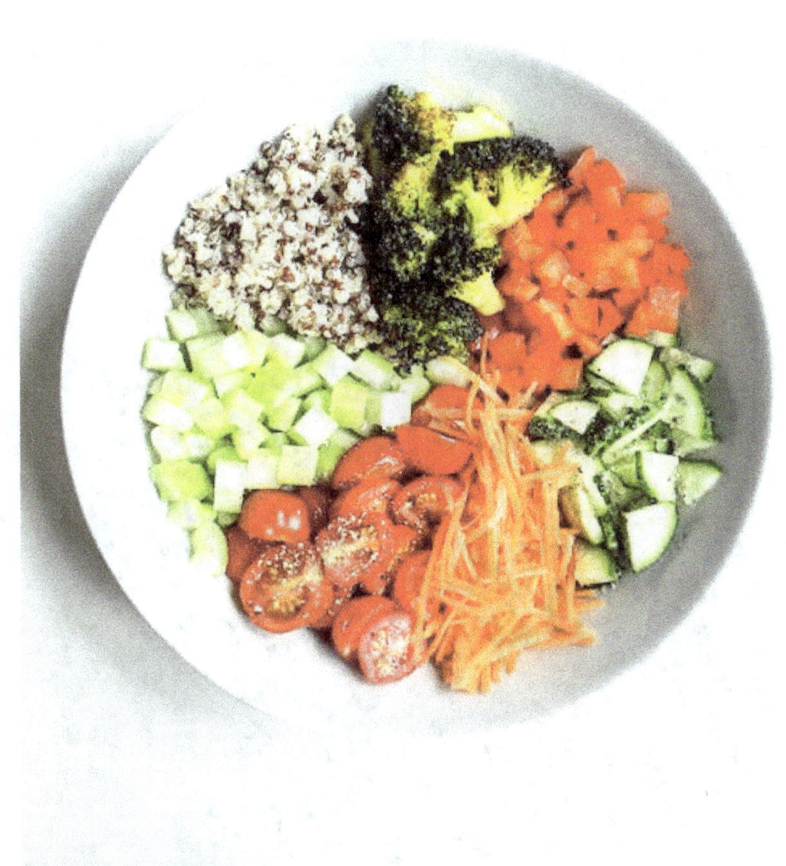

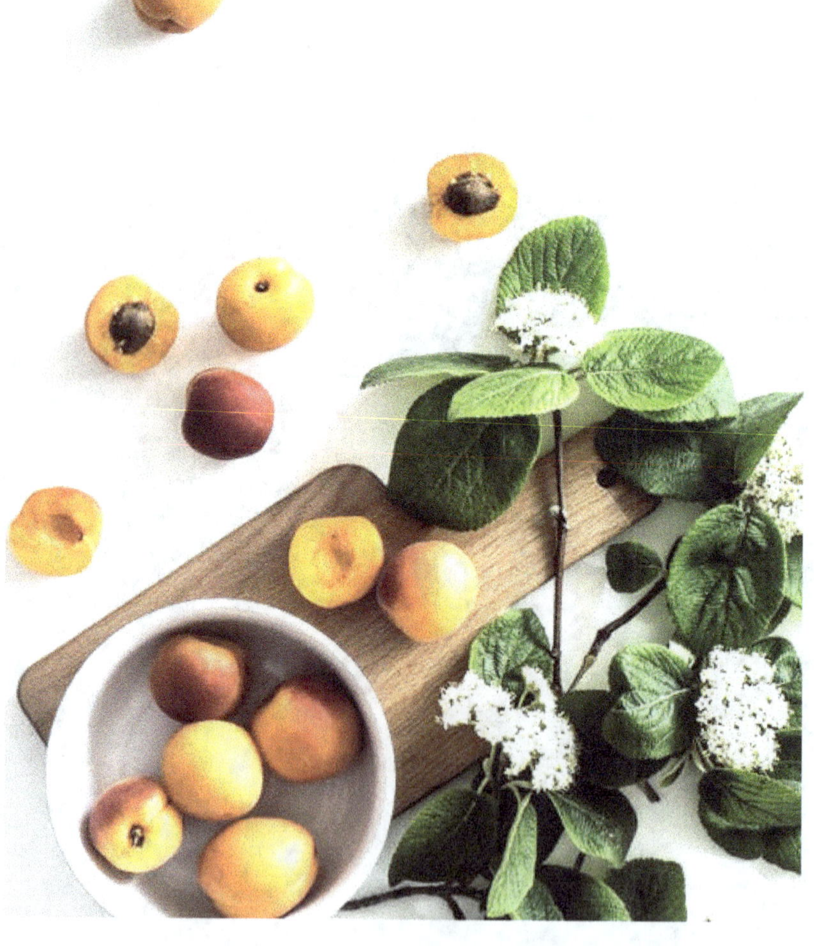

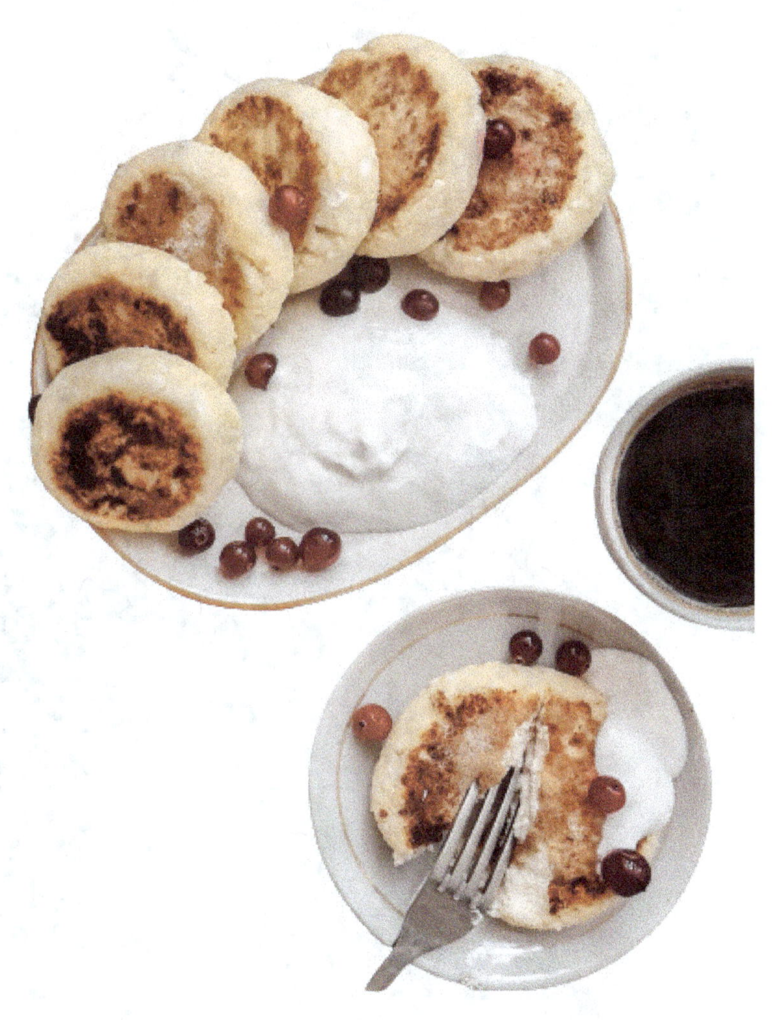

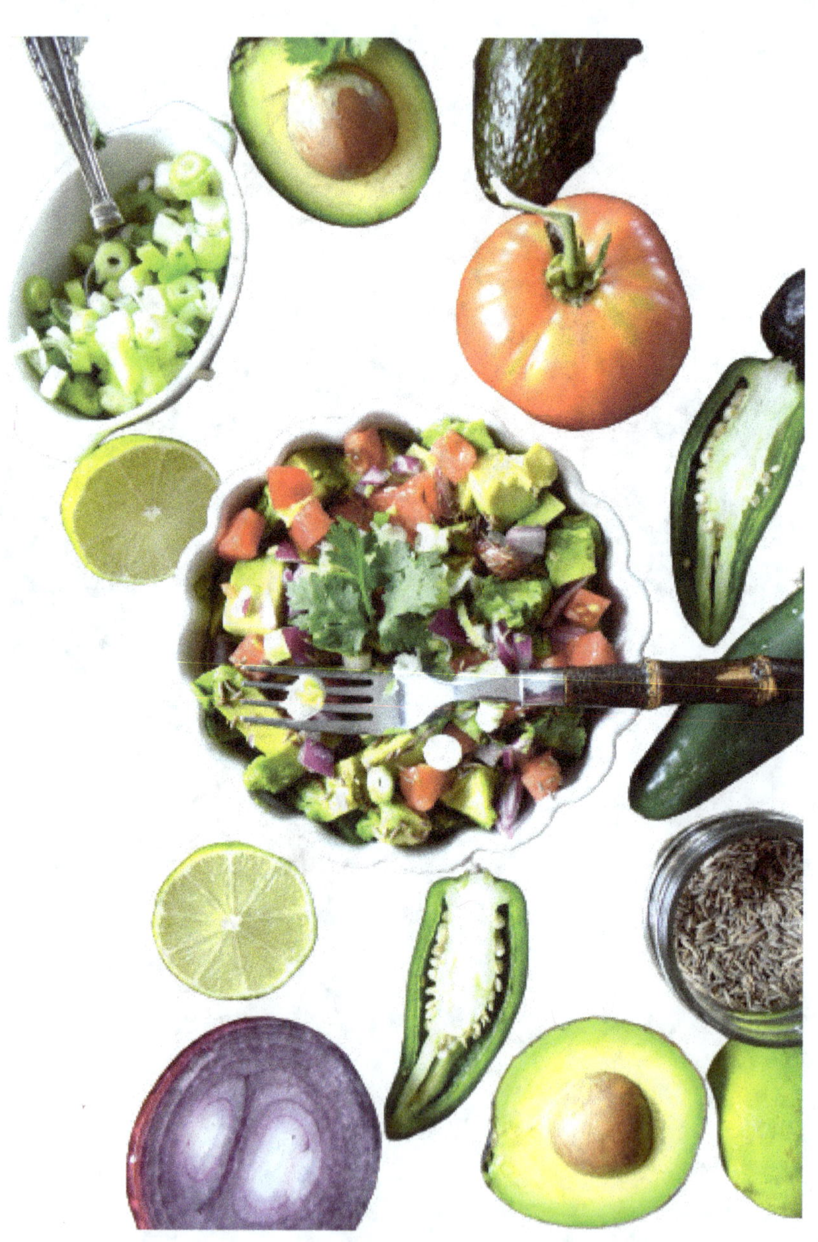

9 798498 234199